1

Table of Contents

Lyme disease is an illness caused by borrelia bacteria. Humans usually get Lyme disease from the bite of a tick carrying the bacteria.

Ticks that can carry borrelia bacteria live throughout most of the United States. But Lyme disease is most common in the upper Midwest and the northeastern and mid-Atlantic states. It's also common in Europe and in south central and southeastern Canada.

You're at risk of Lyme disease if you spend time where the ticks live, such as grassy, brushy or wooded areas. Taking safety measures in these areas can lower the risk of Lyme disease

BREAKFAST

1. Homemade Breakfast Sausage

Prep Time: 10 Minutes

Cook Time: 10 Minutes

Servings: 12

Ingredients

- 1 & 1/2 pounds ground pork (not seasoned Italian sausage)
- 4 cloves garlic , minced
- 2 tablespoons light brown sugar , packed
- 1 & 1/2 tablespoons finely chopped fresh sage
- 1 & 1/2 tablespoons finely chopped fresh thyme
- 1 1/2 teaspoons kosher salt
- 1 teaspoon black pepper
- 1/2 teaspoon crushed red pepper flakes
- 1/2 teaspoon poultry seasoning
- 1/2 teaspoon smoked paprika

Instructions

1. Place the ground pork, garlic, brown sugar, sage, thyme, salt, pepper, pepper flakes, poultry seasoning, and paprika in a large bowl. Mix until combined. Cover with plastic wrap and place in the fridge for at least one hour (overnight is best if you have the time.)

2. Portion the sausage into 12 equal pieces and form into patties.

3. Place a large nonstick skillet over medium heat. Brown the sausage for about 4 to 5 minutes per side or until an internal temperature reaches 165°F.

4. Serve immediately and enjoy as desired with pancakes, eggs, or as a breakfast sandwich.

Prep Time: 15 Minutes

Cook Time: 45 Minutes

Servings: 8

Ingredients

- 1 tablespoon extra-virgin olive oil
- 1 pound bacon , diced
- 1 medium sweet onion , diced
- 2 links cooked Italian chicken sausage , diced small (the size of peas)
- 6 large eggs , lightly beaten
- 1 & 1/2 cups 4% cottage cheese
- 4 cups shredded hash brown potatoes (I use "Simply Potatoes Shredded Hash Browns" in the refrigerator section for ease)
- 2 cups shredded Mexican blend cheese
- 1 & 1/4 cups shredded white cheddar cheese
- 1/4 teaspoon kosher salt
- 1/8 teaspoon pepper
- finely diced scallions , for garnish

Instructions

1. Coat a 9×13 baking dish with nonstick cooking spray.

2. Heat oil in a large skillet over medium-high; add bacon and cook until almost crispy, about 6 minutes. Drain off fat. Stir in the onion and chicken sausage; sauté until onion is soft and translucent, about 3 minutes. Removed from heat.

3. Transfer mixture to a large bowl. Add in the eggs, cottage cheese, shredded potatoes, cheese, salt, and pepper; stir to combine thoroughly.

4. Spread mixture evenly into the prepared baking dish. Cover tightly and place in the refrigerator overnight.

5. In the morning, preheat oven to 350º F.

6. Remove cover and bake for 45 to 50 minutes until eggs are set and casserole is golden around the edges. Let stand 10 to 15 minutes before cutting. Serve with a sprinkle of diced scallions and enjoy!

7. NOTE: Want to cook and serve it right away? No problem! No need to refrigerate overnight. Just preheat the oven while the bacon is cooking.

Prep Time: 15 Minutes

Cook Time: 45 Minutes

Servings: 5

Ingredients

- 2 cups deli ham , chopped small
- 1/2 cup diced scallions
- 2 & 1/2 cups shredded cheddar cheese , divided
- 10 (8-inch) flour tortillas
- 1 & 1/4 cups half-and-half
- 4 large eggs
- 1/2 teaspoon salt
- 1/4 teaspoon pepper
- 1/4 teaspoon garlic powder
- 1 tablespoon flour
- salsa, sour cream, and extra green onions or cilantro for serving

Instructions

1. Coat a 9×13 inch baking dish with nonstick cooking spray.

2. In a medium bowl, mix together the ham, scallions, and 2 cups of the cheese. Scoop 1/3 cup of the cheese mixture onto each tortilla; roll up and place seam side down in the baking dish.

3. Whisk together the half-and-half, eggs, salt, pepper, garlic powder, and flour. Pour liquid evenly over the tortillas. Cover with foil and refrigerate overnight.

4. In the morning, preheat oven to 350° F. Bake, covered with foil, for 35 minutes. Remove foil and sprinkle remaining 1/2 cup of cheese over enchiladas. Bake for 10 more minutes or until tops are golden brown and the egg mixture is set.

5. Serve with salsa, sour cream, and additional green onions or cilantro.

Prep Time: 15 Minutes

Cook Time: 1hrs 5 Minutes

Servings: 10

Ingredients

- 1 pound ground breakfast sausage
- 1 medium onion , diced
- 1 small red bell pepper , diced
- 2 cloves garlic , minced
- 8 large eggs
- 2 cups milk
- 1 teaspoon garlic powder
- 1/2 teaspoon kosher salt
- 1/2 teaspoon pepper
- 1/2 teaspoon dry ground mustard (optional)
- 1 1/2 cups shredded Colby jack cheese , divided
- 28 ounces frozen tater tots

Instructions

1. Preheat oven to 350 degrees F. Coat a 9×13 casserole dish with nonstick cooking spray.

2. In a medium nonstick skillet, combine the sausage, onions, and bell pepper over medium-high heat. Cook, breaking up the sausage into crumbles with a wooden spoon, until browned and no pink remains. Add in the garlic and cook until fragrant, about 20 seconds. Drain the grease from the sausage mixture and spread it in the casserole dish.

3. In a mixing bowl, whisk together the eggs, milk, garlic powder, salt, pepper, and dry mustard (if using.) Pour the egg mixture over the sausage mixture.

4. Sprinkle half of the cheese and all of the tater tots into the casserole dish.

5. Bake the casserole for 55 minutes. Sprinkle the remaining cheese on the top of the casserole and bake for an additional 5 minutes, or until eggs are cooked through.

6. Let stand 5 minute before serving and enjoy!

7. NOTE: like your food more spicy? Feel free to swap out the breakfast sausage with hot sausage and/or replace the colby jack cheese with pepper jack.

Prep Time: 30 Minutes

Cook Time: 35 Minutes

Servings: 8

Ingredients

- 2 1/2 cups Tater Tot Crowns
- 1 tablespoon extra-virgin olive oil
- 1 pound Italian pork sausage (or sweet breakfast sausage)
- 8 large eggs
- 1/2 cup half n half
- 1/2 teaspoon kosher salt
- 1 1/2 tablespoons unsalted butter
- 1 1/2 cups shredded Cheddar cheese
- 2 whole scallions , diced
- 8 large (10-inch) flour tortillas

Instructions

1. Preheat oven to 400 degrees F. Lightly coat a baking sheet with nonstick cooking spray.

2. Cook tater tots according to package directions.

3. In the meantime, warm olive oil in a large nonstick skillet over medium-high heat. Add the sausage and cook, breaking it up into small crumbles with a wooden spoon, until cooked through and no pink remains. Drain off fat; transfer to a bowl. Wipe out the skillet.

4. Follow these instructions to make your scrambled eggs (which include the half-n-half, kosher salt, and butter.)

5. IF you are eating these right away and NOT freezing them, you'll want to evenly divide and distribute the ingredients into 8 portions down the center of each tortilla: approximately a scant 1/3 cup of the cooked sausage. Top with 5-6 tater tot crowns, 1/3 cup of the scrambled eggs, 2-3 tablespoons of cheese, and a little sprinkle of scallions.

6. Fold in opposite sides of each tortilla, then roll snugly from the bottom up. Place seam side down on the prepared baking sheet.

7. Place into the oven and bake until heated through, about 12-15 minutes.

8. Let stand 2-3 minutes, then eat and enjoy!

9. If you ARE freezing these, see the recipe notes (below)
    for directions.

Prep Time: 15 Minutes

Cook Time: 20 Minutes

Servings: 6

Ingredients

- 4 large eggs
- 1/4 cup half-n-half
- 1/4 teaspoon kosher salt
- 1 tablespoon unsalted butter
- 8 ounce tube refrigerated seamless crescent roll dough sheet
- 3-4 teaspoons mustard
- 8 slices thin deli ham
- 1 cup shredded cheddar cheese or Mexican blend
- chopped fresh parsley, for garnish

Instructions

1. Preheat oven to 375 degrees F. Line a large baking sheet with parchment paper.

2. Beat the eggs with the half and half and salt, then make Scrambled Eggs.

3. Unroll the dough sheet onto the prepared baking sheet. Cut 10 slits (on each of the long sides) about two-thirds of the way in, leaving the center one-third uncut. (Reference the picture in the blog post and watch the video – they help.)

4. Spread the mustard along the center of dough. Top with the ham, scrambled eggs, and cheese. Crisscross the dough strips over the filling so that you get a braided pattern, making sure the filing is secure and the dough adheres to each other.

5. Bake for 20-23 minutes until golden brown (tent with foil after 18 minutes if it's getting too brown.) Remove from oven and sprinkle with the parsley.

6. Let rest for 5 minutes, then slice and serve immediately.

Prep Time: 10 Minutes

Cook Time: 10 Minutes

Servings: 2

Ingredients

- 2 tablespoons STAR Butter Olive Oil, divided
- 1/4 cup diced red bell pepper
- 1/4 cup diced orange bell pepper
- 1 small jalapeño, diced (seeds removed)
- 1/2 cup diced sweet onion
- 2 eggs, beaten
- 3/4 cup colby jack cheese, divided
- 2 (8-inch) flour tortillas
- salt and pepper

Instructions

1. In a large non stick skillet, warm 1 tablespoon of the butter olive oil over medium-high heat. Add the bell peppers, jalapeño, and onion. Saute for 5 minutes until the vegetables are soft; season with salt and

pepper. Add in the eggs, cook, stirring often, until the eggs are just set, about 1-2 minutes. Transfer mixture to a bowl and keep warm.

2. Brush one side of each tortilla with the remaining tablespoon of butter olive oil. On the un-oiled side, sprinkle half of the cheese, the egg mixture, followed by the remaining cheese, and topped with the 2nd tortilla, oiled side up.

3. Clean out the skillet with some paper towels and heat up again on medium-high. Once hot, place the quesadilla in the pan and let cook for a minute; check the underside to see if it's browned and crispy; flip with a large spatula and cook the other side for 1-2 minutes until golden and cheese has melted.

4. Transfer to a cutting board and slice into 8 wedges. Serve with salsa and sour cream, if desired.

Prep Time: 30 Minutes

Cook Time: 15 Minutes

Servings: 2

Ingredients

- 2 naan flatbreads
- 1 tablespoon pesto, divided
- 4 strips bacon, cut into 1/2-inch pieces
- 1/2 cup diced red or orange bell pepper
- 1/2 cup diced sweet onion
- 1/2 tablespoon unsalted butter
- 1 cup Simply Potatoes shredded hash browns (found in the refrigerator section at the market)
- 1 1/2 cups Italian blend shredded cheese
- 1 scallion, diced
- 2 eggs
- salt and pepper

Instructions

1. Preheat oven to 475 degrees. Place oven rack in lowest position.

2. In a large nonstick sauté pan, cook the bacon over medium heat, stirring occasionally, until crispy, about 7 minutes. With a slotted spoon, transfer to a plate lined with paper towels. Add the bell pepper and onion to the pan with the rendered bacon fat and sauté until tender, about 5 minutes; season with salt and pepper. Transfer to a bowl. In the same pan, heat the butter; once melted add in the hash browns and cook, stirring occasionally, until golden, about 7 more minutes. Transfer to a bowl.

3. To assemble the pizzas, place flatbread on baking sheets lightly coated with cooking spray. Spread the pesto evenly on each flatbread. Then evenly distribute the cheese, hash browns, pepper/onion mixture, bacon, and scallions. Move a portion of the toppings out of the way to make 2 little wells (1 on each flatbread.) Crack eggs into the wells. Sprinkle with a little pepper.

4. Bake until the crust is golden and the eggs are set, but still slightly soft, about 15 minutes. Serve immediately.

Prep Time: 20 Minutes

Cook Time: 55 Minutes

Servings: 10

Ingredients

- 2 tablespoons extra-virgin olive oil
- 1 1/2 cups diced cooked ham
- 1 small sweet onion , diced small
- 1 small red bell pepper , diced small
- salt and pepper , to taste
- 2 scallions , diced
- 2 tablespoons chopped fresh parsley
- 15 ounce loaf french or Italian bread , day old, cut into small 1-inch cubes
- 2 cups shredded Colby Jack cheese , divided
- 10 large eggs
- 3 cups half-n-half
- 1/2 teaspoon kosher salt

Instructions

1. Warm the olive oil in a large nonstick skillet over medium-high heat. Toss in the ham in an even layer and don't touch for a minute, to develop a nice crust. Then stir for a minute.

2. Add in the onions and bell pepper; cook until soft, stirring occasionally, about 3 minutes. Season with a little salt and pepper. Remove from the heat and stir in the scallions and parsley. Set aside.

3. Lightly coat a 9×13 baking dish with nonstick cooking spray. Scatter the bread cubes on the bottom. Sprinkle with half the cheese, followed by all of the cooked ham mixture.

4. In a large bowl, whisk together the eggs, half-n-half, and salt. Pour over the top of the casserole; cover and refrigerate overnight. (Bring to room temperature before baking.)

5. Preheat oven to 350 degrees F. Uncover; sprinkle remaining cheese evenly over the top.

6. Bake for about 50-60 minutes or until puffed and golden and a knife inserted comes out clean. Let rest for 10 minutes before serving.

7. Cut into squares and enjoy!

Prep Time: 15 Minutes

Cook Time: 25 Minutes

Servings: 8

Ingredients

- 7 slices bacon , diced small
- 3 tablespoons unsalted butter
- 1 tube refrigerated Pillsbury Grands biscuits
- 3 large eggs , beaten
- 1/3 cup shredded sharp cheddar cheese
- 1/3 cup shredded monterey jack cheese
- 2 scallions , finely diced

Instructions

1. Cook bacon in a large skillet over medium-high heat until crispy, stirring occasionally, about 5 minutes. Drain on a paper towel and set aside.
2. Preheat the oven to 350 degrees F.

3. Put the butter in a nonstick bundt pan coated liberally with cooking spray and let it melt in the preheating oven.

4. While the butter melts, cut the Grands biscuits into quarters. In a bowl, gently toss the biscuit pieces, cooked bacon, eggs, both cheeses, and scallions together.

5. Once the butter has melted, give the bundt pan a little swirl so the bottom is evenly coated. Add the biscuit mixture to the pan, sprinkling with any cheese and bacon pieces that get left behind.

6. Bake for 25-27 minutes or until golden.

7. Run a dull knife around the edges of the pan to loosen. Turn out on a dish and enjoy!

11. Broccoli Cheddar Soup

Prep Time: 15 Minutes

Cook Time: 25 Minutes

Servings: 6

Ingredients

- 5 tablespoons unsalted butter , divided
- 1 small sweet onion , diced small
- 1/4 cup flour
- 2 cups whole milk
- 2 cups low-sodium chicken broth
- 1 & 1/2 cups coarsely chopped broccoli florets
- 1 large carrot , cut into matchsticks (1 cup)
- 1 stalk celery , thinly sliced (1/2 cup)
- 10 ounces sharp cheddar cheese , shredded (2 & 1/2 cups)
- 3/4 teaspoon salt
- 1/2 teaspoon black pepper
- 1/4 teaspoon ground mustard
- pinch cayenne pepper

Instructions

1. In a large saucepan over medium-high heat, melt 1 tablespoon of the butter; add in the onion and saute, stirring, until translucent, 3-4 minutes.

2. Reduce heat to medium-low and melt the remaining 4 tablespoons of butter. Add in the flour and whisk until dissolved and combined.

3. Gradually add in the milk, whisking constantly until no lumps or flour remain, then whisk in the chicken broth.

4. Bring to a boil, then reduce heat to a gentle bubble, whisking occasionally for 5 minutes.

5. Add in the broccoli, carrot, and celery; gently simmer until vegetables are tender, about 10-15 minutes.

6. Reduce heat to low; stir in the cheese until melted, about 1 minute. Stir in the salt, pepper, ground mustard, and cayenne.

7. Ladle into bowls and serve immediately.

Prep Time: 15 Minutes

Cook Time: 15 Minutes

Servings: 4

Ingredients

For the Tonkatsu Sauce:

- 1/4 cup ketchup
- 1 tablespoon Worcestershire sauce
- 1/2 tablespoon low-sodium soy sauce
- 1/2 tablespoon mirin
- 1/2 tablespoon granulated sugar
- 1 teaspoon brown sugar
- 1/4 teaspoon garlic powder
- 1/8 teaspoon ground ginger

For the Chicken:

- 4 boneless skinless chicken thighs (5 ounces each)
- 1/2 teaspoon coarse salt
- 1/4 teaspoon freshly ground black pepper
- 1 large egg
- 1/2 tablespoon vegetable oil

- 1/4 cup all-purpose flour

- 1 1/3 cup panko Japanese breadcrumbs

- 3 cups vegetable oil , for deep frying

For Serving

- katsu sauce

- cooked sticky white sushi rice

- shredded cabbage salad

- macaroni salad

- sliced tomato

Instructions

1. Make the katsu sauce by whisking all the ingredients together in a small bowl. Taste and adjust the sauce according to your liking. Set aside.

2. Trim any excess skin, fat, or gristle off of each chicken thigh, then place between some plastic wrap and tenderize the meat, gently pounding until both sides are flattened and about a 1/2-inch even thickness.

3. Sprinkle the salt and pepper evenly over the surface of each side of the chicken pieces.

4. Set up a breading station with 3 shallow bowls: one with the flour, one with the egg, and one with the

panko breadcrumbs. (Beat the egg with the 1/2 tablespoon vegetable oil.)

5. Dredge the chicken with a thin coating of flour, making sure not to miss any spots, shaking off any excess. Then coat it in the beaten egg, making sure there is no dry flour left, letting any excess dip off. And finally coat the chicken in the panko fully, gently pressing the panko into the cutlet to adhere.

6. Add the oil to a medium-size, heavy-bottomed pot – the oil should be 1 & 1/2 inches deep. (If you use a larger pot, you will need to add more oil to get it 1 & 1/2 inches deep.) Start heating the oil to 340F over medium heat.

7. Once oil has reached 340F, gently lower one piece of chicken at a time into the hot oil and deep-fry for 3 to 4 minutes on each side, until crispy and golden brown and the chicken is cooked through at 165F. Using tongs, remove the chicken cutlet from the oil and transfer to a paper towel-lined plate to drain off the grease.

8. Using a handheld skimmer, remove any crumbs in the oil and bring the temperature back up to 340F (if it dropped) so it's still bubbling, before adding the next piece of chicken.

9. Allow the chicken to rest for 2 minutes before slicing. Cut the chicken into 1-inch wide strips.

10. Serve with some of the katsu sauce, and a side of shredded cabbage, sticky white rice, macaroni salad, and sliced tomato.

Prep Time: 20 Minutes

Cook Time: 20 Minutes

Servings: 6

Ingredients

For the Dressing:

- 3 tablespoons mayonnaise
- 3 tablespoons plain Greek yogurt
- 2 tablespoons red wine vinegar
- 1 teaspoon lemon juice
- 1/2 teaspoon garlic powder
- 1/4 teaspoon onion powder
- 1/4 teaspoon sriracha hot sauce (optional)
- coarse salt and freshly ground pepper , to taste

For the Salad:

- 8 hard boiled eggs , quartered, then quartered again (so each egg is cut into 8 pieces)
- 6 slices bacon , cooked until crispy, crumbled
- 1 small avocado , cubed
- 1/2 cup cherry , halved crosswise

- 1/3 cup crumbled Roquefort blue cheese
- 2 tablespoons fresh chopped chives
- coarse salt and freshly ground pepper , to taste

Instructions

1. Make the dressing: whisk together the mayo, Greek yogurt, vinegar, lemon juice, garlic powder, onion powder, and sriracha (if using.) Season with a pinch of salt and a couple turns of freshly cracked pepper.
2. In a large serving bowl, lay out rows of the egg, bacon, avocado, blue cheese, and cherry tomatoes. Then gently fold in the dressing to coat.
3. Garnish with chives and just a touch more ground pepper.
4. Serve as a salad on individual plates or bowls (or in lettuce cups as an appetizer.)

Prep Time: 15 Minutes

Cook Time: 25 Minutes

Servings: 6

Ingredients

- 1/2 cup all-purpose flour
- 1 teaspoon garlic powder
- 1 teaspoon salt
- 1/2 teaspoon pepper
- 1 large egg
- splash of milk
- 2 & 1/2 cups sweetened coconut flakes
- 1 & 3/4 pounds chicken tenders , patted dry
- 1/4 cup unsalted butter ,melted
- 1/2 cup apricot jam
- 2 tablespoons Dijon mustard

Instructions

1. Preheat the oven to 400 degrees F. Line a baking sheet with parchment paper; set aside.

2. In a medium shallow bowl, whisk together the flour, garlic powder, salt, and pepper.

3. In a second medium bowl, beat together the egg and milk.

4. Put the coconut flakes in a third shallow bowl.

5. Dredge each chicken tender in the flour mixture, then in the beaten egg (letting any excess drip off), then coat with the coconut mixture, pressing down so the flakes stick. Place on the baking sheet. Repeat this process with all the chicken tenders.

6. After all chicken pieces are coated and on the baking sheet, drizzle them with the melted butter.

7. Bake for about 22 minutes (or until the chicken registers 165 degrees), flipping halfway through cooking time. (At the halfway point, if the coconut is browning too quickly, tent with foil.)

8. While chicken cooks, prepare the apricot sauce by mixing the preserves with the mustard in a small bowl. Keep in the refrigerator until ready to use.

9. Serve chicken with the dipping sauce and enjoy!

Prep Time: 15 Minutes

Cook Time: 15 Minutes

Servings: 6

Ingredients

For the Dressing:

- 1 & 1/4 cups mayonnaise
- 2 & 1/2 tablespoons spicy brown mustard
- 1 tablespoon paprika (sweet or smoked)
- 1 tablespoon parsley , finely chopped
- 2 teaspoons prepared horseradish
- 2 teaspoons lemon juice
- 1 teaspoon Creole seasoning
- 1 teaspoon sweet pickle juice
- 1 teaspoon hot sauce
- 1 clove garlic , grated
- couple turns of freshly cracked black pepper

For the Salad:

- 6 cups chopped romaine lettuce (rinsed and dried)

- 1 pound shrimp , medium sized, cooked and chilled, tails OFF
- 4 large hard boiled eggs (quartered, sliced, or chopped)
- 1 ripe avocado (sliced or chopped)
- 1 cup grape or cherry tomatoes , halved
- 2 tablespoons chopped chives
- kosher salt and freshly ground pepper , to taste

Instructions

1. Make the dressing: Place all ingredients into a jar with a tightfitting lid. Shake vigorously until well-blended and emulsified. Taste and adjust seasonings, adding more salt and pepper if necessary. (Alternatively, you can just whisk everything together in a bowl until incorporated and smooth.) Cover and place in the fridge until ready to use.

2. Assemble the salad: Divide lettuce evenly among 4 shallow bowls. Then top with rows of shrimp (in the middle), hard-boiled egg, avocado, and cherry tomatoes. Garnish with chopped chives and season with a bit of salt and pepper, to taste.

3. Drizzle some dressing over the salad just before serving and allow people to add more, if they like.

Prep Time: 20 Minutes

Cook Time: 10 Minutes

Servings: 16

Ingredients

For The Pretzel Crust:

- 2 1/2 cups finely crushed pretzels
- 3 tablespoons granulated sugar
- 3/4 cup unsalted butter , melted

For The Jello Topping:

- 6 ounce box orange gelatin
- 10 ounce can DOLE Mandarin Oranges , drained, juice reserved and chilled

For The Creamy Filling:

- 8 ounces cream cheese , softened
- 1 cup granulated sugar
- 8 ounces cool whip topping , thawed

Instructions

Make the crust:

1. Preheat oven to 350 degrees F. Coat a 9×13 baking dish with nonstick spray.
2. In a medium bowl, mix together the pretzels, sugar, and melted butter. Press evenly into the bottom of the prepared baking dish. Bake for 10 minutes, or until mixture is lightly toasted. Set aside to cool completely.

Make the topping:

1. In a medium bowl, whisk together the orange gelatin powder with 2 cups boiling water. Stir until completely dissolved. Then whisk in the reserved cold mandarin orange juice. Chill in the fridge for about 1 hour to partially solidify (but not too much longer or it will set too much and you won't be able to pour it.)

Make the filling:

2. In a medium bowl, beat the cream cheese and sugar with a handheld mixer. Fold in the whipped topping until thoroughly combined. Spread evenly over the cooled pretzel layer, making sure it goes completely to the edges so the jello layer doesn't leak through.

3. Evenly place the mandarin orange segments on top. Chill for 30 minutes. Then pour chilled orange gelatin over the cream cheese layer.

4. Refrigerate until completely chilled and set, at least 4 hours (or overnight). Slice and serve!

Prep Time: 10 Minutes

Cook Time: 5 Minutes

Servings: 4

Ingredients

For the Sauce/Dressing:

- 1/2 cup mayonnaise
- 2 tablespoons finely diced sweet onion
- 2 tablespoons ketchup
- 1 teaspoon prepared yellow mustard
- 1 tablespoon sweet pickle relish
- 1 teaspoon white vinegar (or lemon juice)
- 1/4 teaspoon sweet paprika
- 1/8 teaspoon kosher salt

For the Salad:

- Nonstick spray
- 1 pound lean ground beef
- 1 teaspoon kosher salt
- 1/2 teaspoon ground black pepper
- 1/4 teaspoon garlic powder

- 6 cups shredded iceberg lettuce
- 1/2 cup finely diced onions
- 1 cup shredded sharp cheddar cheese
- 1/4 cup finely diced dill pickles
- toasted sesame seeds , for garnish

Instructions

1. Make the dressing: Whisk all the dressing ingredients together. (If it's too thick to drizzle, you can thin it out with just a bit of water.) Set aside while you cook the beef (or cover and refrigerate if using later.)

2. Cook the beef: Warm a large nonstick pan over medium-high heat. Once hot, spray with nonstick spray and add the ground beef. Cook, undisturbed for 1 minute, so it can develop a nice brown color. Then sauté, breaking it up into tiny crumbles, until cooked through and no pink remains. Drain off the fat, then season with the salt, pepper, and garlic powder. Transfer beef to a shallow bowl to cool slightly.

3. Assemble the salad: In rows, divide the lettuce between 4 salad bowls (about 1 1/2 cups each.) Top with about 1/3 cup beef, the cheddar cheese, diced onion, and pickles. Drizzle about 3 tablespoons of the

Big Mac sauce over each salad and toss to coat. Garnish with a little bit of toasted sesame seeds and enjoy.

Prep Time: 20 Minutes

Cook Time: 15 Minutes

Servings: 8

Ingredients

For the Salad:

- 8 ounces dry elbow macaroni pasta
- 6 large hard boiled eggs
- 2 ribs celery , diced small
- 1/3 cup red onion , finely diced
- 2 medium dill pickles , finely diced

For the Sauce:

- 1 cup mayonnaise
- 2 tablespoons dill pickle juice
- 1 tablespoon apple cider vinegar
- 1 tablespoon dijon mustard
- 2 teaspoons granulated sugar
- 1/4 teaspoon salt
- 1/4 teaspoon ground black pepper
- 1/8 teaspoon garlic powder

- 1/8 teaspoon paprika

For Garnish:

- paprika
- diced scallion

Instructions

1. Bring a large pot of salted water to a boil; cook pasta al dente according to package directions. Drain and run under cold water. Set aside.
2. As the pasta is cooking, peel the eggs and separate the whites and yolks. Chop up the egg whites and set aside. Transfer the egg yolks to a large bowl and mash with a fork (or for a smoother consistency, crush them with a wooden spoon into a powder.)
3. To the bowl, add all the ingredients for the dressing. Whisk until combined and smooth.
4. Add in the cooked and cooled macaroni, chopped egg whites, celery, red onion, and dill pickles. Gently stir well until combined. Taste and adjust seasoning if necessary.
5. Just before serving, garnish with a scant dusting of paprika and a sprinkling of finely diced scallions.

Prep Time: 10 Minutes

Cook Time: 10 Minutes

Servings: 8

Ingredients

- 1 teaspoon dried parsley
- 1/4 teaspoon garlic powder
- 1/4 teaspoon paprika
- 1/4 teaspoon salt
- 1/8 teaspoon black pepper
- 1/2 cup unsalted butter melted
- 1 cup Panko breadcrumbs
- 3 tablespoons freshly grated parmesan
- 1 boneless skinless chicken breast

Instructions

1. Preheat air fryer to 390 degrees for 5 minutes.
2. In a small bowl, combine the dried parsley, garlic powder, paprika, salt, and pepper.

3. In another small bowl, combine the melted butter, breadcrumbs, and parmesan.

4. Trim any excess fat from chicken breast. Slice into 1/2-inch thick strips, then each slice into 2 to 3 nuggets.

5. Sprinkle the chicken pieces with the seasoning mixture and then dip each piece into the breadcrumbs, pressing to adhere.

6. Place nuggets in the air fryer basket, in a single layer without touching. (Cook in batches if necessary, depending on the size of your air fryer.)

7. Air fry for 6 minutes, flip them over and air fry for another 3 to 4 minutes. (Check nuggets with a thermometer and make sure they have an internal temperature of 165 degrees F. If not, air fry for a few more minutes. Exact cooking time will vary depending on the size of your nuggets, your air fryer, etc.)

8. Remove nuggets from basket with tongs and set onto a plate to cool.

9. Serve right away with your favorite dipping sauce.

Prep Time: 15 Minutes

Cook Time: 4hrs 10 Minutes

Servings: 6

Ingredients

- 2 pounds boneless skinless chicken thighs , excess fat removed
- 1 ounce taco seasoning (homemade or store-bought 1 ounce packet)
- 1/2 cup salsa
- 4 cups cooked white rice
- 1 cup black beans , drained and rinsed
- 2 cups shredded iceberg lettuce
- 1 cup shredded Mexican cheese
- 1 tomato , diced
- 1/2 cup guacamole
- 1/4 cup sour cream
- 1 lime , cut into wedges, for serving

Instructions

1. Coat a 6-quart slow cooker with nonstick cooking spray. Add the chicken and sprinkle the taco seasoning and salsa over the top.

2. Cover and cook for 4-6 hours on the low setting. (Mine is usually done at 4 hours, but it could take longer. Check for an internal temperature of 165 degrees. You don't want to over-cook the chicken or it will be dry.)

3. Remove lid. Using two forks, shred the chicken into bite-size pieces.

4. Evenly divide the rice into 6 bowls. On top of the rice, evenly divide the chicken mixture.

5. Top the chicken with beans, lettuce, cheese, tomato, guacamole, and sour cream.

6. Served with some lime wedges and enjoy.

Prep Time: 20 Minutes

Cook Time: 1hrs 10 Minutes

Servings: 6

Ingredients

- 2 & 1/2 pounds red or yukon gold potatoes , sliced thin (do not peel)
- 2 tablespoons butter
- 2 cloves garlic , minced
- 2 tablespoons flour
- 1 cup whole milk
- 1 cup heavy cream
- 1 teaspoon salt
- 1/2 teaspoon pepper
- 3/4 cup sharp cheddar , shredded
- 3/4 cup smoked cheddar , shredded
- 1/2 cup parmesan , grated
- 2 tablespoons fresh chopped herbs (parsley, chives, thyme)

Instructions

1. Preheat the oven to 350°F. Grease a 9×13 casserole dish.

2. In a medium saucepan, melt butter over medium heat. Add garlic and cook for 20 seconds. Add flour and cook for 1-2 minutes to make a roux. Slowly whisk in the milk and cream and bring to a boil. Reduce heat to low and whisk in fresh herbs and 3/4 of the cheeses, reserving some for the top.

3. Place a small amount of cheese sauce in the bottom of the pan. Layer with half of the sliced potatoes. Add 1/2 of the cheese sauce and then repeat with another layer of potatoes followed by the remainder of the cheese sauce. Top with the rest of the shredded cheese and cover with foil.

4. Bake for 75-90 minutes, or until potatoes are tender and edges are bubbly. Remove foil and broil until the cheese on top browns (watch it carefully to prevent burning. It can happen fast!)

5. Cool for at least 30 minutes before slicing, to prevent slices falling apart. The sauce will thicken as it cools.

21. Cranberry Buckle

Prep Time: 20 Minutes

Cook Time: 45 Minutes

Servings: 9

Ingredients

For The Topping:

- 1/3 cup all-purpose flour
- 1/4 cup granulated sugar
- 1/4 cup brown sugar
- 1/4 cup cold butter , cut into small cubes
- 1/2 teaspoon ground cinnamon

For The Cake:

- 3/4 cup granulated sugar
- 2 tablespoons shortening
- 2 tablespoons butter , softened
- 1 egg
- 2 teaspoons orange zest
- 1/2 teaspoon vanilla

- 1 & 3/4 cups all-purpose flour , spooned and leveled
- 2 teaspoons baking powder
- 1/2 teaspoon kosher salt
- 1/2 cup whole milk
- 1 & 3/4 cups cranberries (fresh or frozen)

Instructions

1. Preheat oven to 350 degrees F. Grease an 8×8-inch pan.
2. For the topping: Using a fork, pastry blender, or your hands, combine all the ingredients until you have pea size crumbs. Place in the fridge while you make the cake batter.
3. For the cake: In a large bowl with an electric mixer, cream together the sugar, shortening, and butter until light and fluffy. Beat in the egg, orange zest, and vanilla until combined, smooth, and fluffy.
4. In a separate bowl whisk together the flour, baking powder, and salt. Stir into the butter/shortening mixture, alternating with milk, mixing until just combined. (Batter will be thick.)
5. Fold in the cranberries, then spread batter evenly into the prepared pan.

6. Remove topping from the refrigerator and break it up into tiny pieces, then sprinkle evenly over the cake batter.

7. Transfer pan to the preheated oven and bake for 40-50 minutes or until a toothpick in the center comes out clean.

8. Cut into squares and enjoy!

Prep Time: 20 Minutes

Cook Time: 30 Minutes

Servings: 6

Ingredients

- 2 pounds carrots , peeled
- 1/4 cup extra-virgin olive oil
- 1 & 1/4 teaspoons kosher salt
- 1/2 teaspoon freshly ground black pepper
- 1/4 teaspoon garlic powder
- pinch of cracked red pepper flakes
- 2 teaspoons honey
- 2 tablespoons apple cider vinegar
- 1/2 cup toasted sliced almonds
- 1/3 cup dried cranberries
- 4 ounces crumbled feta cheese
- 2 cups baby arugula

Instructions

1. Preheat oven to 400 degrees F.

2. If the carrots are thick, cut them in half lengthwise; if not, leave whole. Then slice the carrots diagonally into 2-inch thick pieces. Place onto a baking sheet, then drizzle with the olive oil and season with the salt, pepper, garlic powder, and cracked red pepper flakes. Toss to coat and then spread them out into a single layer.

3. Roast the carrots in the preheated oven until tender and the edges turn brown, tossing once, about 25 to 30 minutes. Remove and allow to cool to room temperature. Once cool, transfer carrots to a large mixing bowl.

4. Whisk together the honey and cider vinegar; drizzle half of the mixture with the carrots until coated.

5. Add the almonds, cranberries, and feta cheese; toss again until evenly mixed.

6. Combine with the arugula and toss with the remaining dressing, if needed, right before serving so the leaves don't wilt.

Prep Time: 20 Minutes

Cook Time: 4hrs 30 Minutes

Servings: 10

Ingredients

For The Brine (Optional)

- 4 cups water
- 1 cup kosher salt
- 1 cup sugar
- 1 lemon
- fresh or dried herbs also used below (optional, but recommended)
- 1/2 onion (optional, but recommended)
- 3 cloves garlic , smashed (optional, but recommended)
- ice cubes
- 2 gallons cold water

For The Turkey

- 10-14 pound fresh turkey
- 1 teaspoon kosher salt

- 1 teaspoon black pepper
- 4 sprigs fresh rosemary
- fresh sage
- 6 sprigs fresh thyme
- 2 large carrots , peeled and halved
- 2 large ribs celery , halved
- 1 medium onion , peeled and quartered
- 6 cloves garlic , smashed
- 1 lemon , halved
- 3 tablespoons butter , melted
- 1 tablespoons canola oil
- 32 ounces low sodium chicken broth
- additional fresh herbs , for garnish

Instructions

1. If you are using a fresh turkey that has not been injected with saline solution, start the night before with a brine: In a large pot, bring 4 cups of water to a boil, add salt and sugar stirring until dissolved. Add the lemon, herbs, onion, and garlic cloves. Add a few cups of ice to help to cool it down quickly. Place the turkey in a brining bag, add the brine solution and remaining cold water. Brine the turkey overnight in

the fridge. The next day, rinse turkey, pat dry, and bring up to room temperature before continuing with the following steps.

2. Preheat the oven to 350 degrees F. Position oven rack in the middle, or one step lower if needed to fit your turkey. Bring your turkey up to room temperature and pat it dry. Remove the giblets and save the neck if you'd like to use it to fortify a gravy. Place the breast side up on a roasting rack in a large roasting pan. Season the turkey inside and out with the salt and pepper.

3. Squeeze the lemon halves on and inside the turkey. Place half the herbs, garlic, lemon, and onion in the cavity, and place the other half in the roasting pan with the celery and carrots. Fold the wings under the back and tie the legs together with some kitchen twine, this ensures a more even roasting process. Mix together the butter and oil, and brush liberally on the turkey.

4. Pour about half of the chicken broth in the bottom of the pan.

5. Roast the turkey for 15-20 minutes PER POUND or until an instant read thermometer inserted into the thickest part of the breast without touching the bone

reads 165F, and the juices run clear from the cavity.
(Cover loosely with foil if the turkey starts browning
too fast. Add more broth as needed to keep the bottom
of the pan moist.)

6. Remove the turkey from the oven and tent loosely
   with foil – the temperature will continue to rise as it
   rests. Rest turkey for at least 15-30 minutes before
   carving. Save pan drippings if you want to make a
   gravy.

Prep Time: 15 Minutes

Cook Time: 30 Minutes

Servings: 6

Ingredients

- 4 tablespoons salted butter
- 1/4 cup granulated sugar
- 1/4 cup packed light brown sugar
- 1 teaspoon ground cinnamon
- 2 & 1/2 pounds Golden Delicious apples , peeled and cored, 1/2 inch slices (see note below)
- 1/2 cup apple juice
- 1 tablespoon + 1 teaspoon cornstarch

Instructions

1. In a large skillet over medium heat, add the butter, sugar, brown sugar, and cinnamon. Stir constantly until the butter and sugars are melted.
2. Add the apples and coat them in the mixture. Place a lid on the pan and bring it to a simmer. Simmer for

15-20 minutes until crisp-tender, gently stirring every few minutes.

3. In a bowl mix together the apple juice and the cornstarch. Slowly stream this into the simmering apples, stirring constantly. Cook for one minute until thickened.

4. Serve immediately and enjoy!

Prep Time: 15 Minutes

Cook Time: 30 Minutes

Servings: 6

Ingredients

For the Meatballs:

- 1 pound lean ground beef
- 3/4 cup panko bread crumbs
- 1 large egg
- 2 teaspoons ketchup
- 1 teaspoon dijon mustard
- 1 teaspoon garlic powder
- 1/2 teaspoon dried oregano
- 1 teaspoon kosher salt
- 1/2 teaspoon freshly ground black pepper
- 2 tablespoons extra-virgin olive oil (for the skillet)

For the Gravy:

- 2 tablespoons unsalted butter
- 2 tablespoons flour
- 1 & 1/2 cups beef stock

- 1 tablespoon ketchup
- 1 teaspoon Worcestershire sauce
- 1/2 teaspoon onion powder
- salt and pepper , to taste

For Serving:

- 8 ounces freshly shredded melty cheese (such as gruyere, provolone, or mozzarella)
- 6 hoagie rolls
- Fresh finely chopped thyme or parsley

Instructions

1. In a large bowl, mix all meatball ingredients with your hands (except the oil) until just combined.
2. Using a cookie scoop, shape the mixture into 1 & 1/2-inch balls (about 2 tablespoons each) rolling briefly between the palms of your hands.
3. Place on a clean platter, cover and refrigerate for about 30 minutes, if possible – this helps them retain their round shape when cooking.
4. In a large nonstick skillet, warm the olive oil over medium-high heat until shimmering. Working in batches to avoid crowding, add the meatballs and

cook turning continuously until browned on all sides, about 5-6 minutes (reducing the heat if they're browning too much.) Repeat with the remaining meatballs. Transfer to a plate and cover with foil.

5. Reduce the heat to medium and in the same skillet with the drippings, add the butter. Once melted, add in the flour and whisk constantly until combined and no lumps remain.

6. Slowly pour in the beef stock, whisking well. Add in the ketchup, Worcestershire, onion powder, whisking to combine; bring to a simmer, then turn down the heat to a gentle bubble and let the sauce thicken, stirring continuously for about 2 minutes. Season with salt and pepper, to taste.

7. Add the partially cooked meatballs back to the skillet and nestle into the gravy; cover and cook another 8 to 10 minutes until cooked through (with an internal temperature of 160 degrees F.)

8. Assemble the Sandwiches

9. Slice open the hoagie rolls and place under the broiler on low until they are light golden brown (watch very closely so they don't burn!) OR just put them in the oven to get crisp and golden.

10. Arrange 3 meatballs on one side of each hoagie, top with a handful of shredded cheese, broil (or bake) on low until the cheese is melty.

11. Garnish with a little finely chopped fresh thyme or parsley and serve immediately.

Prep Time: 15 Minutes

Cook Time: 20 Minutes

Servings: 6

Ingredients

- 2 tablespoons extra-virgin olive oil
- 1 medium sweet onion , diced
- 3 cloves garlic , minced
- 1 pound lean ground beef
- 1/2 teaspoon kosher salt
- 1/4 teaspoon crushed red pepper flakes
- a few turns of fresh cracked black pepper
- 2 tablespoons tomato paste
- 2 cups low-sodium chicken broth
- 2 cups marinara sauce
- 2 cans (15 ounces each) diced tomatoes , undrained
- 1/2 tablespoon Worcestershire sauce
- 2 teaspoons Italian seasoning
- 1/2 teaspoon paprika
- 1 & 1/2 cups macaroni pasta , uncooked
- 3/4 cup shredded cheddar cheese

- 1/4 cup chopped fresh parsley

Instructions

1. Heat olive oil in a large dutch oven or pot over medium-high. Add onion, garlic, and beef; cook until browned and no pink remains, breaking up into crumbles, stirring frequently, about 3 minutes. Season with the salt, red pepper flakes, and black pepper. Drain excess fat.
2. Stir in the tomato paste until combined.
3. Poor in the chicken broth, marinara sauce, diced tomatoes (with their liquid), Worcestershire, Italian seasoning, and paprika. Season with a bit more salt and pepper, to taste.
4. Bring to a boil and add in pasta; cover, reduce heat to a gentle simmer and cook until pasta is tender, about 14 minutes, stirring occasionally.
5. Remove from heat. Stir in the cheese and parsley.
6. Serve immediately, garnished with additional cheese and parsley, if desired.

Prep Time: 10 Minutes

Cook Time: 20 Minutes

Servings: 4

Ingredients

- 1 pound Brussels sprouts , cleaned, rough outer leaves removed, ends trimmed, halved lengthwise.
- 2 tablespoons extra-virgin olive oil
- 1/2 teaspoon kosher salt
- 1/8 teaspoon cayenne pepper (optional, but recommended)
- 1 cup thinly sliced apple pieces
- 1/3 cup pomegranate seeds/arils
- 1/4 cup chopped pecans
- 1 tablespoon honey
- 1 tablespoon apple cider vinegar
- freshly cracked black pepper , to taste

Instructions

1. Preheat oven to 400 degrees F. Coat a large baking sheet with nonstick cooking spray.

2. Place Brussels sprouts on prepared baking sheet. Drizzle with the olive oil and sprinkle with the salt and cayenne pepper; toss to coat. Then arrange them in a single layer, flat sides down.

3. Place in the oven and cook for 15 minutes.

4. Stir in the apples; place back in the oven for another 5-10 minutes until the Brussels sprouts are crisp-tender and lightly charred.

5. Whisk together the honey, apple cider vinegar, and a couple turns of black pepper.

6. Remove Brussels and apples from the oven and toss with the chopped pecans, pomegranate arils, and honey/cider vinegar.

7. Serve right away and enjoy!

Prep Time: 10 Minutes

Cook Time: 10 Minutes

Servings: 6

Ingredients

- 1 pound dry orecchiette pasta (or short pasta of your choice)
- 2 tablespoons extra virgin olive oil
- 1 small sweet onion , finely diced
- 2 cloves garlic , minced
- 1 pound sweet Italian sausage links , casings removed
- 1/2 teaspoon dried oregano
- 1/8 teaspoon cracked red pepper flakes
- salt and freshly ground pepper , to taste
- 15 ounce can diced tomatoes , undrained
- 1/2 cup low-sodium chicken broth
- 3/4 cup frozen sweet baby peas , thawed
- 1/3 cup heavy cream
- freshly grated Parmesan , for serving

Instructions

1. Bring a large pot of salted water to boil. Cook the pasta to al dente texture, according to package instructions.

2. In the meantime, heat the olive oil in a large nonstick skillet over medium-high heat. Add the onion and sausage; sauté, breaking up the pork into small pieces with a wooden spoon, until no pink remains and the onions are softened, about 4 minutes. Add in the garlic and cook until fragrant, 20 seconds. Drain off fat. Season with the oregano, the crushed red pepper flakes, and a couple grinds of salt and pepper.

3. Add in the tomatoes (with their liquid) and chicken broth. Reduce heat to a gentle simmer and let cook for 5 or so minutes to thicken a bit.

4. Toss in the peas along with the cream; mix and warm through.

5. Drain the pasta and return to the pot, stirring to combine with the sausage mixture.

6. Ladle into shallow bowls and serve right away with a sprinkle of Parmesan.

Prep Time: 20 Minutes

Cook Time: 10 Minutes

Servings: 6

Ingredients

- 6 chicken thighs , bone-in, skin on
- 4 cloves garlic , minced
- 1/2 teaspoon paprika
- 1/2 teaspoon chili flakes
- 1/2 teaspoon garlic powder
- 1/4 teaspoon salt
- 2 tablespoons olive oil
- 5 tablespoons butter
- 1/2 cup chopped onion
- 3 tablespoons lemon juice , freshly squeezed
- 1 tablespoon Italian seasoning
- 1 tablespoon lemon zest
- 1/3 cup low-sodium chicken broth
- 1 tablespoon cornstarch
- 1 tablespoon water

For garnish:

- Fresh chopped parsley and Lemon slices

For serving:

- rice or noodles with a side of roasted vegetables.

Instructions

1. Combine paprika, chili flakes, salt and garlic powder; rub the seasoning onto the skin of the chicken.
2. In the Instant Pot with the sauté function, add 2 tablespoons of olive oil.
3. Add chicken thighs and cook on each side for 2-3 minutes until the chicken is golden brown. Remove chicken from the Instant Pot and set on a plate.
4. Add butter to the instant pot. Add the chopped onion and minced garlic. Sauté for a minute. Add the lemon juice and deglaze the pan by scraping the bits off the bottom. Add Italian seasoning, lemon zest, and chicken broth. Stir to combine.
5. Put the chicken back into the Instant Pot. Put the lid on and lock. Turn the valve to sealing.
6. Set to cook for 7 minutes. When the pressure cooker is done, allow to naturally release for 5 minutes.

7. Turn the valve to release and allow all the steam to release. Push stop.

8. Unlock the lid and transfer chicken to a clean plate and set aside.

9. In a small bowl, whisk together cornstarch and water. Add slurry to the juices in the Instant pot. Turn back to sauté. Whisk and heat until the sauce thickens, about 5 minutes. Put chicken back into the pot, coating with the sauce.

10. Serve and enjoy!

Prep Time: 5 Minutes

Cook Time: 25 Minutes

Servings: 6

Ingredients

- 19 ounces refrigerated tortellini
- 2 cups diced ham
- 1 & 1/2 cups heavy cream
- 2 cups freshly grated parmesan , divided
- 1/2 teaspoon garlic bouillon base (or fresh minced garlic)
- 4 tablespoons butter
- 1/2 teaspoon cinnamon
- 1/2 cup reserved pasta water
- salt and pepper , to taste
- fresh chopped parsley , for garnish

Instructions

1. In a dutch oven or heavy bottomed pot, boil water and cook tortellini according to package instructions.

2. While pasta is cooking, melt butter in a large saucepan over medium-high heat, then whisk in garlic bouillon base and cinnamon. The butter sauce will begin to thicken and bubble.

3. Add the chopped ham, heating it through and browning it slightly on all sides.

4. Drain the tortellini, reserving 1/2 a cup of pasta water.

5. Slowly add the pasta water and heavy cream to the saucepan. Cook for 3-4 minutes, stirring occasionally and de-glazing the bottom of the pan as you go. Season with salt and pepper to your taste.

6. Once the sauce has thickened, remove from the heat and gradually add 1 & 1/2 cups of finely grated parmesan cheese to the saucepan and stir until melted and fully combined.

7. Add in the cooked tortellini and gently toss to coat.

8. Sprinkle on the remaining 1/2 cup of parmesan cheese and chopped parsley. Serve right away ansd enjoy.

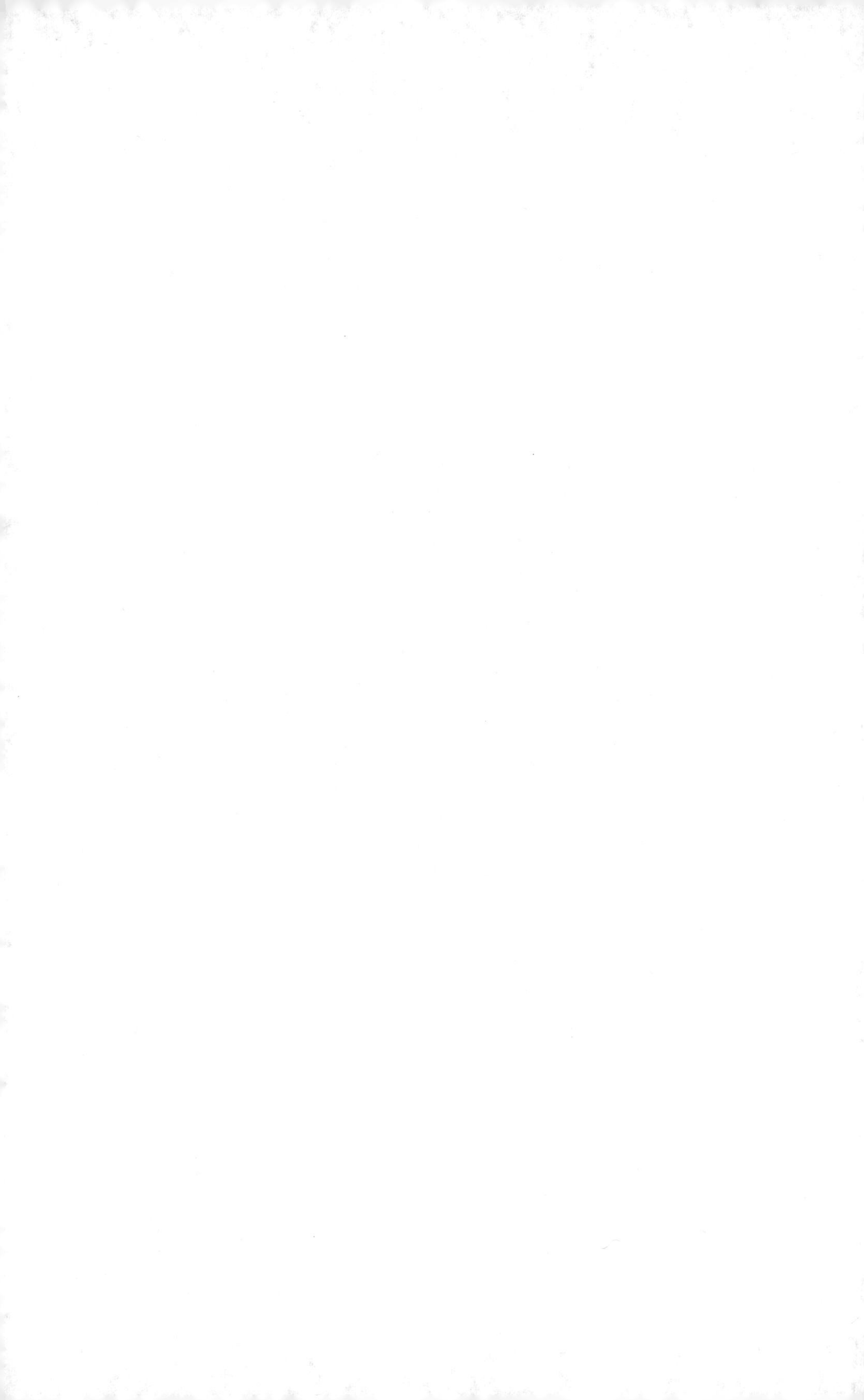